ISBN 9798553083908

CONTENTS

INTRODUCTION

Thank you for buying my book. It is my belief that the information within these pages will be of great value to you. By following my method, it is entirely possible for almost anyone to dramatically reduce the misery of the common cold by up to 99% with a similar level of reduction of the impact that a cold can have on your well-being, not just once, but for all future colds. As far as I can ascertain, my approach differs from any other currently available. It is easy to follow and highly effective. I feel morally obliged to share this information. It is my hope that as many people as possible can look forward to a future where the symptoms of the common cold are reduced to almost zero as a direct result of self-administering a short course of my drug-free therapy.

I feel obliged to point out that I am not a doctor, nor do I have any medical training, however, I consider this to be an advantage because I am free from the constraints imposed by a formal training. This freedom has enabled me to develop a remedy for the common cold that comes very close to a cure. I have developed the remedy described in this book using myself and my wife as 'human guinea pigs'.

As every human body is unique and the common cold can be caused by any one of over 200 viruses, needless to say I have not been able to test the efficacy of my remedy on all of them. Whilst I have personally enjoyed relief of up to 99% from the symptoms of the common cold, it is possible that some people will not gain the same level of relief. Some microbes may either not respond, or respond less well to the regime detailed herein. It is also possible that if you do not get the desired result, you may be suffering from some other ailment and not the common cold, and you should seek advice from your doctor.

1. THE COMMON COLD

The common cold can be caused by any one of over two hundred viruses which may explain why not all colds produce the same symptoms. Personally, I cannot remember having a cold that did not start with a sore throat and until recently I assumed that this was the same for everybody. This assumption was reinforced by all of my family members having had the same experience.

This large number of viruses, most of which are classified as Rhinoviruses and Coronaviruses, that cause the symptoms referred to as the common cold, are the most likely reason why we humans are unable to develop an immunity in order to protect ourselves from further infections. For the same 200 reasons, modern science is currently unable to produce a vaccine and probably never will. Normally a vaccine protects against a single virus, so how can it be possible to protect against so many different viruses? For the same reason there is, not now and probably never will be, a cure. My book does not claim to offer a cure for the common cold, however by following my guidelines you may expect to dramatically reduce the symptoms by up to 99%.

It is thought that the common cold has been infecting people for as long as there have been humans on our blue planet. Fortunately, it is not, in itself, a killer disease although in rare cases it can lead to pneumonia. It can also result in the congestion or mucous getting into the ears or sinuses where a bacterial infection can develop, very likely leading to pain. Persistent or severe infections may require treatment with a course of antibiotics.

I am quite sure, in view of the fact that you are reading this book, that you are very well aware of the symptoms of the common cold and how they affect you as an individual, and that you are looking for an effective treatment. Look no further, you have found what I believe to be the most effective cold remedy on the market, possibly the ultimate.

Every cold causes nasal congestion for the simple reason that the nasal cavity is the main breeding ground for the viruses, triggering our body to response by producing copious amounts of mucous. Following on from that there is a varied menu of other possible symptoms which include sore throat, cough, headache, body aches, high temperature, tiredness, blocked nose, runny nose, sneezing and an overall sense of feeling 'under the weather' and desperately wanting to feel well again.

Then there is the 'dessert menu' of side effects which includes disturbed sleep, sore nose, blocked and painful sinuses, pressure in the ears and an enduring cough.

Unfortunately, we are not able to choose from these menus, we get whatever we are given by the alien invader.

All of these variables, plus the fact that each human is an individual, must surely account for why, to some people, the common cold is a minor inconvenience. For others, it is much more debilitating with some people getting influenza-like symptoms.

I am unable to think of any other illness that affects us as often or as many times as the common cold!

On average, an adult suffers the misery of a cold three times a year. We even give them a variety of names: winter colds, summer colds, head colds etc. We also frequently blame colds on our actions, for example, going outdoors with wet hair or sitting in a draught. In reality, it is a simple matter that a virus has gained access to your body, most likely via your face, as this is where the viruses find the moist and warm environments that they require in order to multiply.

Now for some more bad news….

According to my calculations by the age of eighty it is entirely possible that one may have suffered the unpleasant symptoms of the common cold around two hundred times. This may sound like an impossible number, so here is the fact-based formula that enabled me to arrive at this rather shocking number. Statistics indicate that the average number of times that a child can have a cold is between six and eight per year, while for adults the average is two or three per year.

My rather conservative calculation is as follows:
Six a year for the first ten years creates a sub-total of sixty.

Two per year for the next seventy years gives a second sub-total of one hundred and forty.
Add the two sub-totals together, this makes a total of two hundred.

The bad news gets even worse….

Even more shocking is how much of your life will be spent nursing a cold. Assuming that the symptoms of each cold lasts for just one week, again a **very conservative estimate,** then by the time you are eighty, you will have spent FOUR YEARS of your life suffering the misery inflicted by the common cold.

If I now adjust my calculations as follows:
Six colds per year up to the age of 10,
Three colds per year between the ages of 10 and 80
Adjust the duration of the symptoms to 10 days
The result is 2,700 days or 7 years and 5 months.

What a waste!

Waste no more of your life suffering the misery of the symptoms of the common cold as my book will explain how you may achieve a reduction of symptoms by up to 99%.

2.   THE GOOD NEWS

Some illnesses are avoidable. The polio vaccine has virtually eliminated this horrible disease. The MMR vaccine has had much the same effect on measles, mumps and rubella. But can there ever be a vaccine for the common cold with its multitude of causal viruses?

In view of the fact that antibiotics do not kill viruses, there will, almost certainly, never be a cure. Unless you enjoy the symptoms of the common cold, which I very much doubt, you will be pleased to read that I have developed a drug-free treatment which **reduces all of the symptoms by up to 99%.** This means that the common cold could now be added to the list of avoidable illnesses, or more correctly, avoidable symptoms.

The remedy detailed in this book is so effective at reducing the symptoms, that it enables me to confidently state that you may never again need to suffer the symptoms of the common cold. It is also very simple. In fact, it is so simple that I cannot imagine why it took me so long to develop and why nobody else has arrived at the same conclusion.

Even if antibiotics were able to effectively combat the common cold, using them would not come close to offering a 99% reduction of the symptoms for a very simple reason. By the time that the cold symptoms have developed sufficiently for you to require a doctor's appointment, the cold symptoms would already be at their peak. You may then have to wait for an appointment with your doctor. Then assuming that antibiotics could have an impact on the viruses, which they cannot, it could be several more days before you start to feel better. The remedy proposed within these pages is capable of denying the cold viruses any possibility of evolving into a fully developed cold. In other words, provided that you follow my instructions, starting at the first sign of a cold, you should be able to continue with your life as normal with absolutely minimal symptoms.

If I were to tell you, at this point, that the actual duration of a cold is three to five days you would probably say that I, the author, am talking a load of rubbish.

We all know that a cold lasts considerably longer than that, don't we?
The truth is that a cold really does only last for three to five days depending on the causal virus and your body's immune system response. It is actually the symptoms which can continue for a much longer period of time. This is where my remedy is highly effective. It stops the viruses in their tracks, kills them in vast quantities, thus denying them any possibility of making your life a misery.

Provided that you follow my instructions for administering the entirely natural anti-viral agent, starting as early as possible then, and only then, can you really expect to reduce all of the symptoms of a cold to almost zero. Recovery time is also virtually eliminated as opposed to the weeks or months that an untreated cold often requires.

While there are many ways, both ancient and modern, for reducing each of the symptoms of the common cold individually, my method harnesses one element of the earth's bounty, enabling you to reduce **all** of the symptoms to almost zero.

There is no mystery attached to my remedy. No need to change your lifestyle. No requirement to exercise. No drugs of any sort.

In order to cure a cold, it would be necessary for modern science to develop or discover an agent that is capable of killing the viruses, all 200 + varieties of them!
There are just two elements required for my remedy to be effective.
An anti-viral agent or virucide combined with an effective method of application.

In order to bring about the level of relief from the symptoms of the common cold that I have experienced, it is necessary to employ a virucide. Killing as many of the viruses as possible is the only way that you can hope to get a 99% reduction of the symptoms.
So, what is this drug-free virucide?

The answer is silver.

Do not be dissuaded by comments from health professionals stating that there is no evidence that silver kills viruses as, quite simply, they will be contradicting themselves. Silver is used for the manufacture of some surgical instruments because it guarantees that the instrument remains virus-free, due entirely to silver's natural ability to kill all known viruses and bacteria on contact. Because silver is entirely natural, it can be used safely and is therefore unlikely to have any side-effects for the majority of people.

Silver is being used increasingly in the manufacturing and pharmaceutical industries.
I will list just a few;

Socks to combat odour.
Face masks to kill viruses.
Wound dressings (plasters) to speed healing by keeping the wound sterile.
Mattresses to control bacteria and therefore odours.
Coatings on certain medical instruments and implants to defeat pathogens.

For those of you who are unfortunate enough to be allergic to silver, please do not put this book to one side or throw it away. There are some suggestions for you towards the end of this book. Almost every other detail is the same for you, so please continue to the end.

Nature has provided us with silver which is extremely effective at killing viruses. However,

putting an object made of silver in your mouth is not going to be a great deal of help. It is vital that the silver makes contact with the areas where the viruses are setting up home in your body. Fortunately, there is a product called Colloidal Silver, which, when used according to my instructions, makes it possible for the silver to contact and kill the viruses.
In simple terms, Colloidal Silver is water and micro particles of silver.

My method uses Colloidal Silver which is readily available and easy to administer. Whilst Colloidal Silver is well known for its ability to kill all-known viruses on contact, it requires a system of application for it to be effective up to 99%. My book explains the simple and highly effective technique that I have developed and improved over a period of more than twenty years. Following the simple steps described below may enable you to obtain up to a 99% reduction of the symptoms of the common cold. My remedy is, to the best of my knowledge, different from any other currently on offer.

3. THE BACKGROUND

Before I describe my (possibly) unique method of administering Colloidal Silver I would first like to explain why it is an ally, when used sensibly, and not an enemy or a danger as some people would like you to believe.

There has been a certain amount of scaremongering concerning the use of Colloidal Silver, so let me put your mind at rest. The negative comments usually state that the use of silver causes skin discolouration. This **was** true many years ago, however in reality these comments relate to early experiments using photographic silver in high doses.

These experiments were abandoned following the discovery of penicillin. Unlike photographic silver, (Silver Bromide etc.) Colloidal Silver is produced by the use of low voltage electricity to infuse water with a small amount of pure silver.

As a result, Colloidal Silver consists of just two entirely natural ingredients, without any chemical processes, chemical additives, or preservatives. The result is not a true solution but more a suspension of extremely small particles of silver.

The silver particles are so small that they are invisible to the naked eye. This gives the impression that what you are looking at is simply water, crystal-clear spring water.

I can honestly and categorically state that **occasional** use of Colloidal Silver over a period of more than 20 years, treating the symptoms of the common cold and other minor ailments, has not caused even the slightest change to my skin-colour, despite having consumed multiple litres.

Colloidal Silver is not a new product, it has been commercially available for at least 40 years. Silver has been used as an antiseptic and to protect drinking water for at least 4,000 years.

The Romans knew the value of silver as a means of keeping stored water from deteriorating, even though they had not the faintest idea of how or why it was effective. Nor did they have any notion of the existence of microbes. They threw silver coins into stored water in the belief that the Gods protected their precious water in return for their offerings. Modern science has established that it was in fact the silver and not the Gods that kept their water from deteriorating.

It was more than 20 years ago, having read about the effectiveness of Colloidal Silver at killing microbes that I purchased my first bottle and started experimenting on myself.

Shortly after purchasing my first bottle there was a rather different event that proved to me just how highly effective Colloidal Silver is at killing bacteria. This came in the form of a lower molar toothache whilst I was on holiday. Unfortunately, I had not taken my solution on holiday with me. However, there was a health food shop nearby that stocked it. Having purchased a bottle, I started using it as a mouthwash, holding the solution in the area of the pain for about one minute and then swallowing. This, after several treatments gave me a great deal of relief, to a point where I no longer needed pain killers. I continued with the treatment until I was able to visit my dentist on returning home. An x-ray revealed that the tooth had split in two from tip to root and would need to be removed, so it was hardly surprising that bacteria had entered the split and were causing me pain.

When I was in hospital for a hernia repair, a nurse asked to look at my navel the evening before the operation. At the time this seemed a very odd request, although post operation it was clear why. One of the entry points for the keyhole surgery was very close to my navel.

I am ashamed to say that my navel was somewhat reddened and contained some clothing lint, this needed cleaning before undergoing surgery the following morning. Since having toothache on holiday, I am more inclined to have Colloidal Silver with me when I am away from home and, fortunately, I had taken some into the hospital with me.
I laid down on my back and put 2 or 3 drops of Colloidal Silver directly into my navel. After allowing it to penetrate for a minute, I removed the debris from my navel with a cotton bud and applied another drop of Colloidal Silver. The following morning, I awoke to find that my navel looked 100% clean and healthy and it easily passed the second inspection by a nurse.

More recently I had a bruised sensation at the root end of an upper molar. This I thought was either the start of a toothache or possibly an abscess. A gentle probing with my fingers indicated that the problem was in my sinuses. Shortly before going to bed I used Colloidal Silver as a mouthwash followed by the nasal spray and eye drops. The following morning the sensation was almost completely eliminated, proving to my satisfaction that the Colloidal Silver had indeed entered the sinuses and killed the infection.

When, sometime later, I experienced the bruised sensation on the same tooth for a second time, I naturally assumed that the same treatment would be equally effective. I administered the Colloidal Silver as I had previously, just before going to bed. Sure enough, the following morning there was a great improvement, however, after 23 hours the sensation returned. The following two evenings I repeated the treatment, each time the outcome was the same, that is 23 hours after each treatment, the bruised sensation had returned.

You may not be surprised to learn that I rose to the challenge and changed to a twice daily, morning and evening routine. This treatment regime was still not fully successful, so I increased the number of treatments to three per day at as near to eight-hourly intervals as possible. By following this routine for several more days the discomfort was completely eliminated. The extended time taken to eliminate the infection enabled me to experiment with the method of application of Colloidal Silver. I concluded that the nasal spray on its own was fully effective.

I have included this snippet of information in the hopes of encouraging you to be prepared to adapt and adjust when using Colloidal Silver for purposes other than treating a cold. If you do not feel that you are getting the desired results, it may be prudent to try a modified approach.

Please note that the advice above **does not apply** *to treating the common cold. I have spent more than 20 years developing and improving my method and I am confident that, when you follow my instructions precisely, it is very likely that you will be truly amazed at the outcome.*

I find Colloidal Silver to be extremely effective when used as a mouthwash. Recently, after brushing my teeth, I noticed that my gums were bleeding. A single treatment using Colloidal Silver as a mouthwash proved to be sufficient and the problem has not reoccurred. Unlike other forms of mouthwash, I swallow the solution and do not spit it out. Swallowing the silver solution reduces the risk of the silver staining your wash basin. *Please read carefully the section relating to silver staining, under the heading CAUTION.*

When I was growing up, there was an expression used to describe wealthy people. The person in question was said to have been 'born with a silver spoon in his or her mouth'. It is very likely that wealthy families would have owned and used solid-silver cutlery. As silver is a relatively soft metal it wears away during normal use (as is evident with old silver-plated cutlery where the base-metal can clearly be seen) this enters the digestive systems of the user. Could this be one of the reasons why, in many cases, wealthy families enjoy better health?

When stainless-steel cutlery became readily available and affordable, I changed my silver-plated cutlery in favour of stainless-steel. I presumed that this would eliminate the need to polish the silverware. It is easy to say now, but this may well have been a serious mistake on my behalf!

The real 'danger' with Colloidal Silver, when used in conjunction with my method of application, is that it is so effective at reducing the symptoms of the common cold that one can easily forget that one has a cold and discontinue the treatment too soon, potentially allowing the microbes to resurface. I cannot stress sufficiently the importance of reacting as soon as you possibly can, after detecting the first symptom that a cold is starting. You should continue the treatment for 3 to 5 days.

You may, by now, be wondering if the silver has a negative effect on your gut flora. I have personally never experienced any evidence of a negative impact in this area, leading me to wonder if the silver only kills the 'bad guys' and not the 'good guys.'

The internet offers plenty of information on many subjects including Colloidal Silver. As with any other search you are going to find both positive and negative comments. Please be aware that some authors, for whatever reason, may be biased against Colloidal Silver.

During a recent search, I discovered some seriously conflicting comments:
1. Colloidal Silver is only slightly more toxic than drinking water.
2. The particle size of the silver is so small that it easily passes through our bodies.
3. Colloidal Silver is not harmful to our gut flora (something that I had already thought to be the case).
4. Colloidal Silver will kill you.

I cannot image where this last comment has originated! I am still alive and well after consuming multiple litres of Colloidal Silver over a period of more than 20 years. I am currently 73 years old and consider myself to be in good health. I do not take a single medication, prescribed or otherwise, not even pain killers. If any deaths had been attributed to the use of Colloidal Silver, you can be absolutely certain that the production and sale of it would have been banned long ago. Additional proof is that there are now many more producers and users of Colloidal Silver than there were when I made my first purchase.

I can only recount my own very positive experiences and presume that the negative comments have been posted by well-meaning people who have not given it a fair trial. I fully accept that Colloidal Silver is not a cure-all and make no claim to that effect. However, it has been my experience that it is extremely effective at killing viruses on contact.

The way in which Colloidal Silver kills the viruses denies them any possibility of developing resistance or of mutating. Silver and viruses are attracted to one and other by electricity, rather like rubbing a balloon and using it to lift hair. Once contact is made, the virus is destroyed, but the silver continues its quest unchanged.

Personally, I have complete confidence in Colloidal Silver, both in terms of it being safe to use and its ability to destroy viruses.

You will also find websites offering products or methods that promise a reduction of the symptoms of the common cold. I have been unable to find a single one that proposes a reduction of 99% of the symptoms. To the best of my knowledge, my method of application is unique and differs from any other that I am aware of.

When I first started experimenting with Colloidal Silver to treat the common cold, I only hoped that I would be able to achieve some reduction of the symptoms for myself and my wife. Not even in my wildest dreams did I anticipate that I could achieve a 99% reduction in the symptoms, nor could I have imagined that I would be writing a book aimed at helping other people to avoid the symptoms of the common cold. When I ultimately arrived at the point where I was getting a 99% reduction I was absolutely delighted and just knew that I had to share this information.

The basic principle of my method of application is 'seek and destroy', something that Colloidal Silver does naturally with a high degree of efficiency. My method makes it possible to administer the Colloidal Silver in such a way that enables it to contact as
many of the viruses breeding grounds as possible, resulting in an almost total elimination of their population.

The treatment which is detailed below is the result of more than 20 years of trial and improvement, using myself as a human guinea pig. I now feel confident that I can share this treatment, and that I can state that it offers up to 99% relief from the symptoms. I do not think that it is possible to achieve 100% for two reasons.
The first reason is that a cold has an incubation period, during which time the viruses are quietly multiplying before we experience any symptoms, resulting in the viruses having already established a foothold in our bodies.
The second, I rather think, is that due to the complex form of our internal head cavities, it is likely impossible for the remedy to reach every corner. This may well also provide an explanation as to why the cold will resurface if you stop the treatment too soon. Our bodies' immune response to the alien invasion will destroy the small number of viruses that cannot be contacted by the solution during the 3 to 5-day normal duration of a cold.

One of the reasons why I embarked on the journey that ultimately brought me to the point where I felt compelled to publish this information is that, for many years, I have endeavoured to be my own doctor for minor ailments. My reasoning being that it is inevitable that I know my own body better than anyone else. Whilst I have a great deal of respect for doctors, who spend seven years learning their craft, we, the patients, spend very little time in their company. I would not, in any case, bother a doctor to tell him or her that I have a cold.

I seem to have an in-built ability to look at things in a different way to others. Even as a teenager my father used to say that if there were two ways of doing something then I would find a third and if there were three ways of doing something then I would find a fourth. I have employed this ability in my quest to reduce the symptoms of the common cold.

I also have a stubborn refusal to accept certain things as being inevitable or untreatable and the symptoms of a common cold fell into that category, so I set about finding a way of reducing the negative impact that the common cold would have on my life. I could not have been more pleased at the outcome of my trials. Now I want to share this information, in the sincere hope that it will change a great many lives for the better. For me, one of the worst things about a cold, apart from the obvious symptoms, is that for me and my wife, the most likely time for a cold to strike would be whilst on holiday – not an ideal holiday companion!

I have endeavoured to use straightforward language throughout and to make this remedy as simple as possible so that anyone can follow it. However, it does require a degree of dedication in order to achieve the desired results. Just carry in your mind how unpleasant a cold can be and this will help to remind you to carry out the steps as per the instructions included within these pages. After all, what is three to five days of remembering to follow my instructions as compared to the days of misery caused by the common cold followed by weeks or even months until you feel fully recovered?

I have several vivid memories of times when I felt thoroughly miserable as a result of the symptoms that a cold inflicts, and I now wish that I had made this discovery sooner. I clearly remember having a sore throat that, at the time, seemed unbearable. On one occasion many years ago, my throat felt as though it was on fire, which resulted in me throwing the packet of throat lozenges across the room as they did not seem to be offering any reduction of the pain, particularly when swallowing. We do not realise how often we swallow in response to our body's continual production of saliva until we have a raging sore throat.

Whilst suffering a cold on another occasion, I remember having a nasal cavity solidly blocked with mucous, making it impossible to breathe, other than through my mouth, which only served to make the sore throat even more painful. I also remember the difficulty involved in trying to eat, whilst at the same time breathing through my mouth.

Then there is the sore nose, constant efforts to clear the nasal mucous invariably leads to a nose which is both sore and reddened. In fact, we often comment that somebody has a cold based purely on the redness around his or her nose. I can also remember the discomfort of congested sinuses following a cold which produced a thudding sensation in my face when walking and which elevated to a level rather like an internal thunderstorm when trying to run.

Using my treatment system now offers me the prospect of the rest of my life free from these symptoms. In fact, free from every single one of the symptoms of the common cold. Now you have, in your hands, the information that will enable you to remove these unpleasant symptoms from your life. You simply need to follow my uncomplicated instructions.

Even before I learned about Colloidal Silver, I had already endeavoured to reduce the awful symptoms inflicted by the cold viruses. I would dramatically increase my daily consumption of vitamin C in conjunction with a diet of fresh fruit.

I have read that some of the foods that we all eat on a daily basis are largely responsible for the production of mucous, an excess of which is a major symptom of a cold. Making these changes did bring about a modest reduction of the symptoms, but not enough to stop me from looking for a better alternative.

For most of my adult life, more than 40 years, I have added a good quality multivitamin and mineral supplement plus high strength vitamin C to my diet on a daily basis. I once read that a goat with the same body weight as a human manufactures 5 grams of vitamin C each day and that we humans have long since lost that ability. I have experimented with different doses of vitamin C over the years and find that 5 grams per day is **my** ideal. Any less, or none at all, and I feel tired all day and less able to function well.

I have repeatedly proved to myself that I need vitamin C. As for multi-vitamin and multi-mineral supplements, I consider them as an insurance policy for my health, despite some health professionals stating that they have no value and one might as well take a placebo.

I know that I cannot compare the benefits of taking them with not taking them as I only have one life. However, I can state that I feel well, and take no medication, not even pain killers. I am currently 73 years old and I am well aware that almost all of my friends, all of whom are younger than me, are regularly taking one or more medications and not taking any vitamin or mineral supplements! Could there be a connection?

When I first started experimenting with Colloidal Silver in an attempt to reduce the symptoms of a cold, I only had a bottle of the solution at my disposal and I used this as a gargle and mouthwash before swallowing. This certainly provided some relief, but nowhere near the 99% which I now find achievable. During the years that followed, I added a pump spray, then a nasal spray and finally eye drops. Each addition helped to further reduce the unpleasant cold symptoms.

Once I had all four dispensers available, I would treat the symptoms as they arrived, probably because, when I had a cold prior to using Colloidal Silver, I would have started with throat lozenges, moving on to umpteen boxes of tissues and frequently some form of decongestant. Eventually, and often in desperation, I would have taken some form of cough medicine in an attempt to put a stop to a stubborn cough.

I have experienced, following numerous colds, a cough that has persisted until the summer, after a winter cold. I have also heard other people comment that they have a stubborn cough following a cold.

Without the benefit of any experience, I would administer the Colloidal Silver by gargling and using the pump spray on day one to treat the sore throat. Day two as the congestion developed, I would add the nasal spray and in the event that my eyes became sore I would apply the drops.

This routine brought about a further improvement in the level of relief but still not close to 99%. However, once I started using **all four** methods of treatment, as detailed below, at the first sign of a cold starting, the result truly amazed me, as it produced a level of relief that enabled me to completely forget that I had a cold.

4. THE METHOD

Colloidal Silver – Nature's virucide

You absolutely NEED to buy your colloidal silver BEFORE the first signs that a cold is developing, as even a few hours delay in starting the treatment will inevitably lead to a reduction in the level of relief. Therefore, I recommend that you purchase this essential item at your earliest convenience.

I have avoided making any specific recommendations regarding which brand of Colloidal Silver to buy. This is because I am not affiliated to any other business and the information within these pages is entirely independent and free from any external influence. I can honestly state that I am not in receipt of any form of payment or commission from any third party.

Colloidal Silver is produced in different potencies shown as PPM (parts per million) and may at first seem confusing. My own preference is for a rating of 30 to 45 PPM. The brand that I frequently choose has a stated shelf-life of approximately 3 years.

This does, of course, mean that in the event that you have purchased your stock of Colloidal Silver and have not had the symptoms of a cold, then you are prepared for the following cold season, eliminating the need to make a fresh purchase for the following year. Do however, store your solution in a cool and dark place (maybe even in the fridge, although when the need arises to start using the solution, you might prefer that it is at room temperature). ALWAYS replace the bottle screw tops and the plastic covers of the sprays as soon as possible after use. Failure to do so will allow air to circulate and may cause the silver to oxidise.

I have bought Colloidal Silver at various times in the range of 20 to 80 PPM from a variety of suppliers, including the one that uses clear bottles (more about that later). All have been both genuine and effective. My preference for 30 to 45 PPM is simply because it falls roughly in the middle of the range.

You will need to purchase Colloidal Silver (referred to elsewhere in this book as 'silver solution' or 'solution') in 4 different containers.
A bottle (at least half a litre)
An atomiser spray (pump spray)
A nasal spray
A dropper bottle

Colloidal Silver can be sourced from most independent health food or Bio shops or from the internet, with some suppliers offering a 'bargain bundle' of 3 items.

In order that you do not waste your time searching in the wrong places, I can inform you that, at the time of going to press, both a well-known health food chain and most chemist shops, rather shockingly do **not** stock Colloidal Silver. This information was checked at the time of 'going to press'.

Why so many different dispensers? My own experiences clearly demonstrate that you need to use all four methods of application to reduce the symptoms. However, maximum reduction of the symptoms can only be achieved by using all four dispensers immediately following the onset of a cold.

Consider the complex form that exists inside our heads. Any basic diagram of the internal form of the human head will illustrate just how many cosy corners are available for the viruses to live and breed, with the ultimate aim of making your life a misery.

Colloidal Silver has a distinctive metallic taste which may seem a little unpleasant at first, especially as you will be coating the internal cavities of your head, which, almost certainly will have never experienced the taste of silver. It is my experience that the metallic taste is massively less unpleasant than the symptoms of the common cold! In fact, on a scale of 1 – 10 and placing the cold symptoms at 10 then, for me, the metallic taste of silver is at less than1.

Three things for you to consider, if you find the taste of silver unpleasant, are as follows:
- The metallic taste confirms that the Colloidal Silver is genuine.
- The taste assures you that it is making contact where it is most needed and that it is effectively killing the microbes in vast quantities. Ironically, the areas where we experience the sense of taste and smell are also the areas where the viruses start breeding before they move on to wreak havoc in other areas of our bodies.
- With continued use, your body will become somewhat accustomed to the taste, rendering it less noticeable.

In the unlikely event that you find the metallic taste of silver totally unacceptable, please see my suggestion at the end of this article.

Over the years I have purchased numerous bottles of Colloidal Silver and have never been sold any Colloidal Silver that is not genuine. However, in view of the fact that it looks exactly like crystal clear water, sooner or later some trickster will decide that this a source of easy money. Purchasing from a reliable supplier is recommended and you can easily verify that the product you have purchased is genuine by its unique metallic taste.

5.   INSTRUCTIONS FOR USE

The instructions detailed below may, at first, appear a little complicated. In reality they are quite straight-forward. I have endeavoured to cover every detail so that you will get the maximum reduction of symptoms, starting with your next cold, and also so that you will be able to avoid making the same errors that I made during the 20+ years that I spent developing this remedy.

Use the contents of the **bottle** as a mouthwash and gargle. In addition to gargling you should move the solution around inside your mouth with the intention of rinsing as much of your mouth as possible, including between your teeth, keeping the solution in your mouth for as long as possible before finally swallowing – I find that 10 to 15 millilitres (2 to 3 teaspoons) is an adequate dose.

Swallowing the solution will be of some help in treating your throat. Equally importantly, by not spitting it out, you will reduce the risk of the silver staining your wash-basin. If you have any concerns about swallowing the solution, you can of course, spit it out, however be careful to avoid staining. More about staining later on.

If you use a proprietary mouthwash on a regular basis, it may be a good idea to suspend this activity for the few days that you are using Colloidal Silver. This is simply to eliminate any possible risk of a reaction that might reduce the effectiveness of the silver.

The **atomizer spray** enables you to coat and protect or treat your throat and airways. Point the sprayer into your open mouth and pump as you inhale strongly through your mouth, thereby drawing the spray mist into your throat and airways. I find that 15 to 25 sprays is an effective dose, depending on whether you are using it to protect or remedy.
I have found that the most efficient way of carrying out this part of the remedy is to take multiple short sharp inhales, each one accompanied by a spray of solution.

This method is more effective than trying to pump several times whilst inhaling at the normal rate. I usually manage five short sharp intakes of air, each one accompanied by a spray of the solution, as a replacement for a normal continuous inhale.
It is not possible to give a precise number of sprays to use as individual spray dispensers deliver varying amounts of the solution.

I would like to mention at this point that whilst Colloidal Silver kills the viruses that are the cause of your sore throat and prevent it from getting any worse, there is no possibility that it can repair any damage that has already been caused. The healing process will take time. This is one of the reasons why I stress that you should take action as soon as you notice the first symptoms of a cold. I have proved to myself on numerous occasions that coating my throat before it has become sore and continuing for 3 to 5 days prevents the soreness from developing.

The **nasal spray** is dual purpose. Colloidal Silver is extremely effective at killing viruses on contact. It also works well as a nasal decongestant.

Clearing the mucous is an important step to enabling the solution to make contact with the viruses breeding in your nasal cavity, an area that is difficult to treat in any other way. To the viruses, our nasal cavities must be the equivalent of a spacious luxury hotel in a glamorous resort with superb weather and fine-dining and no bill at the end of their stay! Once they have checked in, their method of breeding leads to a population explosion into unbelievable numbers, triggering the body's defences, including all that yucky mucous that we humans spend time and effort trying to evacuate. It seems to me that the more mucous we evacuate, the more our body produces, leading to a never-ending cycle of congestion and attempts to clear the mucous, resulting in the inevitable sore nose.

Applied correctly, Colloidal Silver changes a billionaire's playground for the viruses into the most inhospitable place imaginable. Colloidal Silver means certain death to the viruses that it comes into contact with, therefore it is very important, even vital, to use the nasal spray, even if you find it a little unpleasant.

Despite the possibility that you may find the taste of silver to be a little unpleasant at first, stick with it, as it would be easy to underestimate its value. After the first few applications you may well notice that it is less unpleasant as the cavities inside your head get used to the taste of silver.

If your nasal cavity is clear apply several sprays into each nostril whilst holding the other nostril closed, at the same time breathing in through your nose so that you draw the solution inwards to where it will be most effective.

In the event that your nasal cavity is already congested, it will be necessary to flush it out, this can be achieved by three or four sprays in each nostril. Hold the solution in place for as long as possible until the mucous has softened and then clear this into a paper tissue. Repeat as many times as necessary until your nasal cavity is clear and then spray several more times into each nostril, this time the aim is to coat as much of the nasal cavity as possible.

It may also be a good idea to re-spray each time after blowing your nose. Once the mucous is ejected, the viruses are more vulnerable to the anti-viral action of the solution. As mentioned above, you need to spray whilst inhaling through your nose to draw the solution inwards.

Properly applied, the nasal spray will also protect your sinuses.
It is possible that you might experience a build-up of mucous in your nasal cavity

during a night's sleep. It is absolutely essential to clear this mucous first thing in the morning and then re-spray, otherwise you risk the viruses getting the upper hand, thereby reducing your ability to enjoy the maximum level of relief from the symptoms.

Gravity dictates that some of the solution will try to escape via your nose. I find that once I have introduced the solution into my nasal cavities, tilting my head back (as if star gazing or watching aerial fireworks) and a certain amount of sniffing will help to keep the solution where it is most effective, which is, needless to say, preferable to letting the solution escape. If the solution gets as far as your throat you may well feel a little surprised and perhaps experience the need to cough, this is due to a normal protective body function and is in no way a cause for concern. It does, however, confirm that your nasal cavity is as fully treated as you can hope for.

People with a cold often say that their nose is blocked. In fact, the nose is simply a conduit and it is the nasal cavity behind the nose which is blocked and where the viruses are multiplying.

Likewise, when we see someone with a reddened nose, we assume that person has a cold. In reality, it is usually the stage where the person is dealing with the follow-on effects of the cold, as it normally takes more than a couple of days for the nose to become sore.

Always clean the spray nozzle after use by rinsing it with running water and then dry with a clean tissue before replacing the protective cap.

Do not be alarmed when, after some time, you notice that the nozzle of the two spray applicators and the glass tube of the dropper bottle become tinted brown, this is a completely normal phenomenon due to the silver reacting to light and air, in the same way as silver jewellery does. It is not only harmless but is also additional proof that the Colloidal Silver that you have purchased is genuine.

Under no circumstances should you even consider using a salt solution or sea-water spray to clear your nose or as a gargle, in combination with Colloidal Silver.

The reason for this advice is to avoid any possible adverse reaction due to the fact that salt is corrosive to silver. In fact, if you follow my instructions, you will soon come to realise that Colloidal Silver is the only product that you will require in order to combat the common cold and to enjoy up to 99% relief from all of the symptoms.

The microbes' entry point can include your eyes and eye sockets as this is another area that is moist, warm and an excellent breeding-ground for viruses. This is just one of the reasons why we are advised, due to the Covid19 pandemic, not to touch our faces. In my experience the symptoms of a head cold often include sore eyes, this is where the **dropper bottle** is useful. A drop or two in each eye, repeated several times a day will relieve the sore sensation, although prevention is, as always, a better option. Therefore, I strongly recommend that you treat your eyes from the first indication that a cold is developing.

In case you are concerned about putting silver in your eyes, let me assure you that I have done so myself, as has my wife, on numerous occasions with no ill-effects.
You may experience a slight stinging sensation at first, just as you would if you put a drop of water in your eye, and not quite as bad as a drop of your own perspiration getting into your eye. This stinging sensation lasts for just a few seconds and is due to a slight difference in the PH values of our eyes and Colloidal Silver.

I have previously read that Colloidal Silver can be used to effectively treat certain eye infections including conjunctivitis.

This information prompted me to use Colloidal Silver in an attempt to cure a recent minor eye infection triggered by a tiny speck of wood getting into my eye. We use wood pellets in our cat's litter tray. When wet, these pellets return to their previous state of sawdust. It was whilst cleaning the litter tray out of doors on a windy day that a speck of sawdust entered my eye, leading to a mild infection. Once the infection had developed sufficiently for me to notice, I started treating it with drops of Colloidal Silver and it took just 5 days to fully recover.

The few drops of Colloidal Silver that were required cost a great deal less than the cost of driving to the doctor's surgery, let alone the cost of a prescribed medication.
In order to obtain the maximum level of relief from all cold symptoms

I strongly recommend using all four modes of application from the outset and at least two hourly, once you have an indication that a cold is starting. An hourly treatment is more appropriate if the symptoms are advanced, and in the event that you get up during the night, repeat the treatment.

In any case, use the treatment last thing at night (going to bed with a clear nose will enable you to sleep better) and first thing in the morning, in addition to the treatments throughout the day. Continue for 3 to 5 days, longer should you feel the need. Continuing for 3 to 5 days is vital, because if you stop the treatment too soon, the viruses may very well resurface and resume their mission to make your life a misery.

Another reason for stating 3 to 5 days is because, depending on the causal virus, the life-span of its rampage in your body is between 3 and 5 days. In any case, it is best to continue until you feel fully recovered. My remedy is so very effective at reducing the symptoms that it may be difficult to decide when to stop the treatment. If you stop too soon and become aware of any one of the symptoms reoccurring, it is simply a matter of restarting the treatment as soon as you possibly can.

May I remind you at this point that there is no cure for the common cold and that the aim of my treatment method is to reduce the symptoms to the absolute minimum. If your work makes a two-hourly treatment difficult or impossible, just follow my instructions as often as your work schedule permits. After all, any treatment is preferable to none.

Whilst I have stated several times that the optimum time to start the treatment is when you notice the first symptom, it is never too late to start treating a cold using my method, as you will still reduce the symptoms and the duration of the cold, although to a lesser extent.

In the event that your life-style requires you to spend time away from home, then I strongly recommend that you carry Colloidal Silver with you at all times, so that you will be prepared and able to start the treatment at the very first indication of a cold. This is particularly important, even vital, in the event that you suffer from frequent or severe colds. Clearly it is not very practical to carry the above 4 items around with you, however if you have the pump spray bottle with you, you can at least use this as 'first aid' until you return home.

6.   FIRST AID

A modified approach is required for 'first aid'. Begin by spraying 15 to 25 times into your open mouth, whilst inhaling, to draw the solution down into your throat.

Secondly, spray multiple times into your open mouth, whilst breathing through your nose, until you have enough liquid in your mouth for you to be able to gargle and swish it around, do this for as long as possible, then finally swallow.
You can also spray your open eyes, although I personally find the drops to be more effective and easier to administer.

In order to treat your nasal cavity whilst away from home, repeatedly spray the solution into the cupped palm of your hand, then 'snort' the liquid, so that it enters your nasal cavity. Repeat this regime as often as possible, perhaps hourly, until you return home.
Instead of carrying your spray bottle with you as you travel to and from your place of work, you can, of course, keep an additional pump spray bottle at your place of work, assuming that you regularly work in the same place or drive the same vehicle etc.

Now that we have all been made acutely aware of the importance of clean hands as a result of Covid19, it may be helpful for you to know that you can use Colloidal Silver to disinfect your hands, just spray it on generously and use normal hand washing motions until it is fully absorbed.

As I have mentioned Covid19, I will share my thoughts with you. I have absolutely no idea if there is any possibility that my cold remedy can be effective against Covid19. As a precaution, on the few occasions that I have been away from home during the lock down, I have used all 4 treatment methods, as listed earlier, as soon as I have returned home. In the event that I experience the first symptoms of covid19 I will, most definitely, give my Colloidal Silver regime a trial. After all, I will have absolutely nothing to lose and potentially everything to gain.

Please note that my comments relating to Covid19 are simply my own ideas and thoughts that are untried and untested. I consider Colloidal Silver may possibly help at the first signs of symptoms. Colloidal Silver is extremely effective at killing microbes **on contact,** however, extremely unlikely to be effective once the microbes, including Covid19, have entered the lungs or bloodstream.

I was very interested to read a recent report on my news-feed in relation to Covid19. The authorities in Japan are using 'a silver compound' in the form of a fine spray as a disinfectant for their public transport. The report states that the 'silver compound' remains effective for longer than other types of disinfectant. I **must** remind you at this point that

Colloidal Silver **will** naturally darken with exposure to light and air and for that reason it is **not** suitable for use on **any** surface that is likely to become **discoloured or stained**.

Please note that I am not in any way claiming that Colloidal Silver will cure covid19. However, it has been repeatedly reported on radio and television broadcasts that any form of illness will weaken your immune system and leave you more susceptible to Covid19. You now have in your hands the ability to reduce the symptoms of the common cold to almost zero and to fully recover in as little as five days from the onset. At least that is one less illness to negatively impact your health. Even the common cold can reduce your immune system's ability to resist other infections.

I do not recommend my treatment method for small children as they will not have acquired the necessary skills. Also, childhood illnesses often better prepare them for adult life. The good news is, that if your child passes the cold on to you, you can treat your own symptoms, ensuring that you can then concentrate on the needs of your child.

During my research I came across the website of a producer of Colloidal Silver. This particular producer mentions a method of treating the common cold in children. I am not repeating this information for two reasons. Firstly, I have not tried or tested this system of treatment. The proposed method of administering the Colloidal Silver is completely different to mine, a system which would be easy enough to use on even the smallest child without any risk of choking. Secondly, the information may be copyright or protected in some way. I will leave you to do your own research!

7.   INFORMATION FOR PARENTS

PARENTS, PROTECT YOURSELVES

When your child comes home from school with the symptoms of the common cold, it makes perfect sense to protect yourself from the risk of the infection passing to you. You can achieve this by simply following my instructions for reducing the symptoms of a cold. A twice daily, morning and evening treatment should offer adequate protection, as you will kill the viruses before they multiply sufficiently for you to experience any symptoms.

ALLERGY ADVICE

Do **not** use this remedy if you have an allergy to silver, for example, if you suffer a reaction to silver jewellery. However, there may be other options available to you. There is more information later on, in the section entitled "**Alternatives to silver.**"

DISCLAIMER

As every human body is unique and the common cold can be caused by any one of over 200 viruses, needless to say I have not been able to test the efficacy of Colloidal Silver on all of them. Whilst I have personally enjoyed relief of up to 99% from the symptoms of the common cold, it is possible that some people will not gain the same level of relief. Some microbes may either not respond, or respond less well to the regime detailed herein. It is also possible that if you do not get the desired result, you may be suffering from some other ailment and not the common cold.

8.   THE COSTS OF TREATMENT

THE COST OF COLLOIDAL SILVER

The initial cost of purchasing Colloidal Silver may seem quite high. In reality, this is not the case when you consider the following: A litre of Colloidal Silver, at the time of writing, can be purchased for around £30. It is not difficult to spend the same amount of money on a meal in a restaurant. Recently whilst dining in a restaurant I paid over £6 for a litre of sparkling water. This means that the price of Colloidal Silver is about 5 times the cost of that bottle of sparkling water.

HOWEVER, the sparkling water will not have any effect in terms of reducing the symptoms of a cold, whereas a litre of Colloidal Silver should treat 2 or 3 colds. In real terms, the cost of treatment could be as little as £10 per cold!

If this still sounds expensive, I would ask you to consider the following:

How much would you normally spend in total on cold remedies?

In order that your calculation of costs is realistic, you should include all of the remedies that you would normally purchase, plus tissues and any other costs such as loss of income.

There is another cost of the common cold to consider. When you come home with a cold there is always the possibility that you will infect other members of your household. Treating your own symptoms with Colloidal Silver will reduce the risk of you passing the cold on to them. The risk of the other family members catching your cold can be further reduced or eliminated if they, in turn, treat themselves twice a day as a preventative measure.

How much would you be prepared to pay for a remedy that almost completely eliminates the symptoms of a cold?

Colloidal Silver when applied using my method, in my opinion, comes very close to total elimination of the symptoms at a very reasonable cost. The almost complete elimination of the symptoms enables you to continue with your life as normal with no need to take sick leave. For many people this means no loss of income.

What value would you put on <u>not</u> spending 4 years of your life nursing a cold?

Colloidal Silver, when applied as I have explained, gives you a choice. Either you can put a stop to the misery of the symptoms of a cold, starting with your next cold and for the rest of your life, **or** you can be dissuaded by those who claim that it will not work or even go so far as to claim that it is dangerous and decide **not** to follow my advice, whereupon you will continue allowing colds to make your life a misery.

REDUCING THE COST OF COLLOIDAL SILVER

A money saving tip is to refill the smaller dispensers from the larger bottle.
Even greater savings can be gained by buying clean empty spray and dropper bottles. However, these bottles **must not be clear glass,** as it is necessary to protect the Colloidal Silver from the effects of light, with the exception of one producer who has developed a range of colours, however as the majority of producers of Colloidal Silver use brown or blue glass, one of these would seem to be the most logical choice of colours.

The following is an example of the additional savings to be made. Buying a litre of Colloidal Silver plus 3 empty **brown or blue** glass applicator bottles (a nasal spray, a pump spray and a dropper bottle) can cost as little as £30 whereas buying all 4 as filled bottles may cost around double that! When you purchase your stock of Colloidal Silver in small quantities it becomes more expensive, i.e. £200 or more per litre for the Colloidal Silver, just for the convenience factor.

CAUTION:

Even though Colloidal Silver looks exactly like water, any spillage that occurs whilst decanting needs to be immediately and thoroughly rinsed away in order to avoid the risk of stains developing. The silver will darken as it naturally reacts to exposure to light and air, just as silver jewellery discolours. The darkening will occur much more quickly than it does on silver objects due to the minute size of the silver particles.

The following suggestions will help you to avoid the silver staining your surfaces. Keep your lips firmly closed while you have the solution in your mouth. Swallow the solution after washing your mouth. Stand your bottles of Colloidal Silver on a protective mat (coaster, folded tissue etc.)

I have recently had confirmation of my long-held theory that viruses like those that cause the common cold can not only be spread by coughs and sneezes putting droplets into the air and then entering another person's body via the moist areas of the face i.e. the nose, mouth and eyes, but also, and just as importantly, by physical contact with an infected person or object, especially if that contact is later followed by touching one's face. This confirmation came about as a result of the covid19 pandemic and seeing the level of protection required by the amazing health-care professionals and listening to the widely broadcast comments about the many ways that the virus is transferred. It has also made us all aware of the importance of clean hands and of avoiding touching our faces.

It is also interesting for me to note that the two areas from which the scientists take samples for analysis are the back of the throat and the nasal cavity, with at least one specialist stating that these are the areas where the Covid19 virus develops. This is the same area where the microbes responsible for the common cold start breeding. It has also prompted me to think that it may only be at a later stage, when their numbers have dramatically increased that the common cold viruses are able to invade the rest of one's body, possibly carried by the mucous produced as a response to the alien invasion. This may explain why attacking the cold microbes as soon as possible is so successful when using my treatment method and why it enables you to almost completely avoid the early symptoms, the symptoms of a developed cold and the complications that frequently manifest themselves later on.

Earlier I mentioned that the real 'danger' of Colloidal Silver in conjunction with my regime was stopping too soon. I recently proved this to myself. Late one evening I noticed that my throat indicated that a cold was developing. I duly carried out the treatment that I propose in this article and I went to bed. The following morning, I had absolutely no sign of the symptoms of a cold and thinking that in fact it was a 'false alarm' I foolishly did not continue the treatment. However, later that evening I became aware that mucous was building up in my nasal cavities, so once again, I carried out all four parts of my treatment regime, and went to bed. I am pleased to say that I slept well, although by the morning the congestion had built up again.

At this point, I realised that it really was a cold and that I should have followed my own advice! This I did, albeit rather belatedly, which enabled me to suffer only very minor symptoms throughout day two. Day three I awoke with a congested nasal cavity and was unable to breathe through my nose, once again I carried out all four parts of my treatment regime including repeatedly spraying and clearing my nasal congestion into tissues until I was able to breathe normally, at which point I sprayed again.
The same day, after breakfast a friend arrived to assist me with a pre-planned D.I.Y. project. I was very happy that I was able to work on the project for 5 hours, only pausing a couple of times to clear some nasal mucous. This was no more frequently than any other morning at that time of year, in fact probably less often!

Based on my experiences of many years and a great many colds, at this stage of an untreated cold I would have been almost continuously trying to clear the mucous and coughing, which would have interfered with my ability to work.

By lunchtime, the nasal congestion had built up again as I had failed to take a break from my work, in order to administer the Colloidal Silver. Once again, using all four methods of treatment quickly cleared the mucous, leaving me free from any cold symptoms for the rest of the day. Day four was unusually mild for the beginning of March and I spent most of the day in the garden with virtually no cold symptoms. Day five I was back to normal with no residual cold symptoms apart from a small amount of mucous that had built up overnight. This was quickly and easily cleared before breakfast, thanks to the use of the nasal spray.

Quick action, at the first indication of a sore throat starting, meant that I completely avoided this symptom, just a very slight tickle from time to time. Repeatedly treating the nasal cavity with the nasal spray meant that I dramatically reduced the production of mucous which resulted in avoiding a sore nose and the coughing stage.

I would estimate that I used less than a quarter of a box of tissues in total, as compared with the probably six to ten boxes that I would have used during an untreated cold before I 'discovered' Colloidal Silver. Despite making foolish errors in my treatment of this particular cold, I was delighted that I was able to achieve around 95% relief from the normal cold symptoms and my work colleague had absolutely no idea that I had a cold.

Writing the previous section has led me to wonder whether the nasal spray can reduce the morning snuffles, which for many years has required me to blow my nose multiple times during the mornings, particularly during the cooler months. Having now tried it, I am pleased to report that using the Colloidal Silver nasal spray does more than simply reduce the morning snuffles. It stops them completely within a minute or two of administering the solution. A single application seems to have a long-term effect as I have now enjoyed at least two weeks without needing to repeatedly blow my nose in the mornings.

9. ALLEGY ADVICE

ALTERNATIVES TO SILVER

There are several other metals available in the form of a colloid. Many of them have a reputation for killing microbes. I have not tested any of them and therefore I am unable to offer any assurances as to their effectiveness in combating the symptoms of the common cold. In theory any of the following could offer another option to those of you with an allergy to silver or an aversion to its taste, you might possibly try Colloidal Gold, Colloidal Zinc or Colloidal Copper as alternatives.

Colloidal Gold is tasteless. Rather surprisingly Colloidal Gold is reddish in colour.

I am currently taking **Colloidal Zinc** orally in an attempt to improve the condition of my prostate gland and am unable to detect any taste other than that of the water.

Colloidal Copper. Copper has a reputation for killing microbes and has been used for thousands of years for healing wounds and for keeping stored water from deteriorating. **As copper is toxic in high doses it is advisable NOT TO SWALLOW after using it as a mouthwash.**

A useful hint for gardeners
I find that when I exclude sunlight and add off-cuts of copper pipe to my rain-water storage containers, the water remains crystal clear!

Another possible alternative for those of you who cannot tolerate the taste of silver is a 3 in 1 combination of Colloidal Copper, Gold and Silver. My wife bought a bottle of this 3 in 1 Colloid when our local shop had temporarily sold out of Colloidal Silver. I tried tasting this and found that it was virtually impossible to detect the distinctive metallic taste of silver. Once again, I have no personal experience with this triple colloid in relation to treating the symptoms of the common cold, although, in principle, this combination **may** possibly prove effective. Clearly this product should **not** be used by people with an allergy to silver, but may suit those of you who cannot tolerate the taste of silver.

Whilst all of the metals mentioned above possess anti-microbial properties, based on my own experiences, I have complete confidence in the effectiveness of Colloidal Silver as a remedy for the symptoms of the common cold. I therefore recommend Colloidal Silver as your first choice of product, if at all possible.

10. FINAL THOUGHTS

Imagine your body as an island.

Taking action against the viruses that cause the common cold has much in common with a war situation. Imagine yourself as an island nation being invaded by an enemy. If you are prepared for the invasion, you can more easily defeat the invaders on the beaches. If you are not prepared, they will over-run your island, build defensive positions and take control of your entire nation. Once they have secured your island, they will be much more difficult to dislodge.

The major difference between this scenario and the reality of the common cold is that the viruses do not need to bring in reinforcements, they simply breed at an alarming rate, until they have overwhelmed your 'island'.
My method of combating the common cold is similar to this example. Hit the viruses hard and fast as soon as you are aware of their presence, this gives you the greatest chance of defeating them. There may be a few guerrillas that escape your defensive action but their ability to cause damage is strictly limited, as is their anticipated life-span.

The moral of this story is simple.

Ensure that you have a stock of defensive weapons, in this case, Colloidal Silver.

Be vigilant. Keep a look-out for the invading viruses. Then you will be ready to mount your defensive action at the first sign that your 'island' is under attack.

Use all four methods of defence without hesitation.

Continue your defensive action until all of the invaders have perished. This should take between 3 and 5 days, a great deal less than the time normally taken to recover from an untreated cold.

An important reminder

Be sure to buy your Colloidal Silver in advance and remember to take it with you when you are away from home for more than a few hours, particularly when going on holiday. It is an invaluable asset in your first aid kit as it has many more first aid applications than simply treating the symptoms of the common cold! Please feel free to share this information with close relatives. However, if you would be prepared to recommend the purchase of my book to your friends, I would be enormously grateful, and I thank you in advance.

I sincerely wish you a future free from the misery of the common cold.

10. STOP PRESS

GREAT NEWS

Ever since the Covid pandemic became headline news, I have asked myself if Colloidal Silver might possibly be of help in beating this particularly nasty virus.

After two long years of staying at home (most of the time) I actually managed to catch Covid, even though I had been triple vaccinated, as has my wife. At 75 years of age this could have been a disaster. However, to me it was a blessing as it gave me the opportunity to test my theory that Colloidal Silver might possibly be effective against other rather more serious viral health threats than the common cold virus.

At first I thought that I had caught a cold; the early symptoms certainly mimicked a cold. The first indication was a slightly sore throat associated with an unpleasant taste, which led me to believe that it was in fact a cold. I immediately started using the formula described in this book and carried on with my life as normal with very slight cold symptoms.

A few days later my wife fell ill, really unwell. Unfortunately, she is not very good at self-diagnosing and even worse at self 'medicating'. She asked me to perform a Covid test on her, which turned out to be positive. At this point she suggested that I should test myself. I said "ridiculous, it is just a slight cold". She insisted, and I eventually agreed if only to prove her fears unfounded. Much to my surprise I tested positive. This led me to believe that the Colloidal Silver had, at the very least, dramatically reduced the potentially devastating effects of Covid.

My wife, on the other hand, was bed ridden for 96 hours. After this she spent several days feeling rather frail whilst recovering. She had used Colloidal Silver, but only to gargle and only very occasionally, and did not start until she felt unable to continue her life as normal.

My own symptoms continued for about 3 weeks, 2 weeks longer than I would expect any minor cold symptoms to last, the main symptom was a runny nose, nothing more serious than that. All of this has led me to believe that the Colloidal Silver had, at the very least, dramatically reduced the potentially devastating effects of Covid.

A full list of my symptoms follows;
A slightly sore throat (this only lasted 2 hours after starting my remedy).
A somewhat congested nose (I have experienced much worse with the common cold prior to using Colloidal Silver).

Slight feverishness.

Some slight muscle aches (arms mainly)

A slight pain in my neck when rotating my head and a restricted ability to rotate (mainly whilst continuing my DIY project)

A mild pain across the base of my abdomen.

A cough.

Loss of sense of smell, much as I would expect with an untreated cold.

A sense that something (perhaps mucous) was moving in my lungs when I took an extra deep breath or laughed.

Most of the above could be mistaken for cold symptoms, and the muscle aches and pains I mistakenly blamed on some D.I.Y. that I was undertaking at the time.

In my case I used Colloidal Silver almost as per my instructions in the earlier chapters of this book, although I have to confess that I allowed my D.I.Y. to distract me and was less than conscientious with the regularity of the doses. The one thing that I did every time that the mucous built up in my nose was to use the nasal spray repeatedly. This successfully cleared my nasal passages and gave a high level of relief from the unpleasant blocked nose sensation.

My experience with Covid has only served to increase my belief that Colloidal Silver can be used to effectively help our bodies resist this most unpleasant virus. Since the first moment that Covid19 was announced I have been convinced that there is, at the very least, a chance that its devastating effects can be limited by the use of Colloidal Silver. My own experience has only served to increase my confidence in Colloidal Silver and my treatment regime.

As with the common cold, IMMEDIATE ACTION is called for. Based on my own experience with treating the common cold and now Covid, starting the treatment as soon as possible after you notice any signs of feeling unwell, dramatically improves one's possibility of beating the virus. With more than two years' experience, living with and fighting Covid19, there are a number of facts known about this particular 'parasite'.

It is well documented that Covid19 likes moist warm environments such as our lungs, so it makes sense to try and kill the virus while it is still in one's nasal cavity and other moist areas of the head and throat.

Now, I am going to suggest that you purchase a piece of equipment called a Nebulizer. Don't wait until Covid comes knocking on your door, be prepared and make the purchase now. Fortunately, I bought one in advance so that I would be prepared for the day that Covid visited my household. A nebulizer produces an atomised spray, resembling steam, which can more easily be drawn into the lungs.

Now, some months later, we have both had another bout of Covid.

Shortly before we were infected, we had both had a blood test to, amongst other things, determine our bodies levels of Covid antibodies. Mine were very high and my wife's levels were very low. Ironically, I was the first to contract the virus and exactly as before I started my Colloidal Silver therapy as soon as I noticed a slight sensation of a sore throat and an unpleasant taste. Once again, I presumed that it was a cold until a few days later when my wife became ill. Although not as serious as the first time, this second attack has left her with a complete lack of taste or smell.

In my case the symptoms have been fewer than the first infection, although it has taken 4 weeks for my nose to stop running. All of this has strengthened my belief that Colloidal Silver used as described in this book can greatly reduce the negative impact of any virus that starts its attack in the moist areas of our heads.

There is another little-known use for Colloidal Silver and that is to protect your hands from Covid. Used BEFORE entering premises that are not your own home, as you would use an alcohol-based hand gel will give you lasting protection. The water will evaporate leaving behind a minute trace of Silver which offers an extended period of protection, as compared to alcohol which, by its very nature, can only be effective in its liquid state.

Some manufacturers offer Silver impregnated masks. We can achieve this at home by spraying a standard mask with Colloidal Silver and letting it dry before use. Just take great care that the spray does not contact any surfaces that it is likely to stain.

I am very well aware that the scientific community would not accept such limited results as mine. However, my philosophy is that I have nothing to lose by, at least trying, to defeat **any** virus that enters my body via the moist areas of my head.

I would like to make it **crystal clear** that once **any virus** has established itself in one's body, then Colloidal Silver will be **much less effective**. This is because silver kills viruses on contact and once the virus has entered our organs or blood stream, contact becomes impossible.

A final thought.

No matter how many times the covid virus mutates IT REMAINS A VIRUS and as such it is susceptible to silver, the natural enemy of all bacteria and viruses.

REMOVABLE REMINDER PAGE

BRIEF INSTRUCTIONS FOR DRAMATICALLY REDUCING THE SYMPTOMS OF THE COMMON COLD USING COLLOIDAL SILVER

<u>AT THE FIRST INDICATION OF SYMPTOMS OF THE COMMON COLD</u>

USE 10 – 15 ML AS A MOUTHWASH AND GARGLE FOR AT LEAST 60 SECONDS AND THEN SWALLOW

USE THE ATOMISER TO SPRAY INTO YOUR OPEN MOUTH WHILST INHALING STRONGLY IN ORDER TO DRAW THE MIST INTO YOUR THROAT AND UPPER RESPIRATORY TRACT

USE THE NASAL SPRAY TO FULLY COAT YOUR NASAL CAVITY

USE THE DROPPER BOTTLE TO APPLY 1 OR 2 DROPS INTO EACH EYE

****

REPEAT ALL FOUR METHODS OF TREATMENT 2 HOURLY IF POSSIBLE

HOURLY IF YOU WERE UNABLE TO START YOUR TREATMENT AT THE FIRST PRESENTATION OF SYMPTOMS

REPEAT IF YOU GET UP DURING THE NIGHT

CLEAR YOUR NASAL CAVITY FIRST THING IN THE MORNING BY REPEATED USE OF THE NASAL SPRAY

<u>ALWAYS</u> TAKE COLLOIDAL SILVER WITH YOU WHEN YOU EXPECT TO BE AWAY FROM HOME FOR MORE THAN 3 OR 4 HOURS

Might I suggest that you keep this page with your stock of Colloidal Silver, in readiness for your next cold or better still photograph it with your phone so that you will have it with you at all times.